The **Metablolic** **WEIGHT LOSS** **DIET Maze.**

50 Effective Weight Loss Recipes to lose

Weight and Battle Invisible Health Risk

...*Inspired By Dr. Barbara O'Neill*

Written By Barnabas Noah

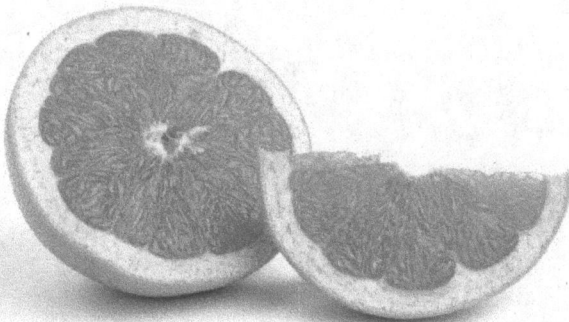

Table of Contents

INTRODUCTION
Welcome to a journey of transformation...

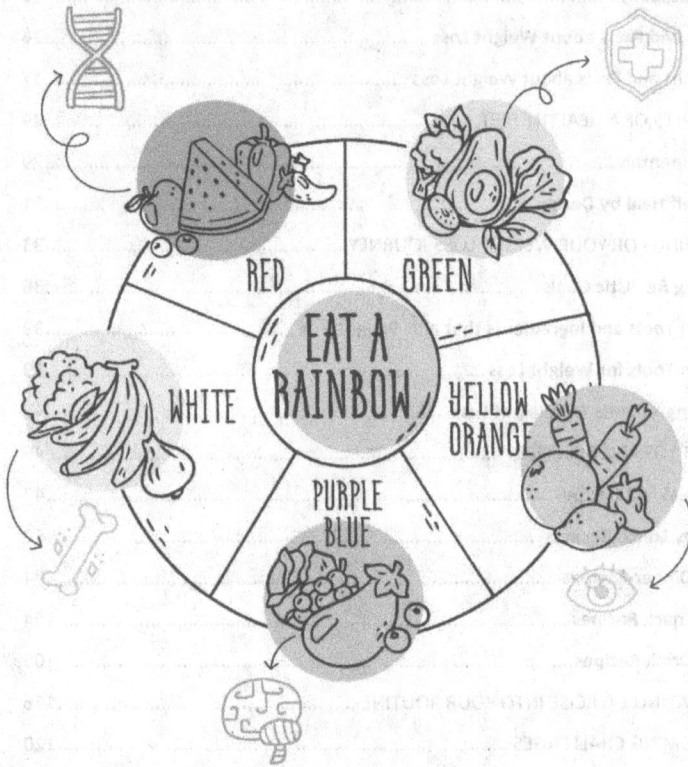

Embarking on a journey towards a healthier, more vibrant you is both exciting and challenging. In this book, "The Metabolic Weight Loss Diet Maze," we will explore the intertwining paths of diet, health, and well-being, all through the lens of natural healing and nourishment. Inspired by the wisdom of Barbara O'Neill and her book "Self Heal by Design," this guide is more than just a collection of recipes; it's a beacon of hope and a testament to the power of natural healing.

The Philosophy of Natural Healing

Barbara O'Neill, a renowned advocate for natural health, has inspired countless individuals to take control of their health through simple, yet profound dietary and lifestyle changes. Her philosophy, rooted in the belief that our bodies have an innate ability to heal and maintain balance, serves as the cornerstone of this book. In these pages, we embrace the idea that food is not just sustenance, but medicine and that making informed, conscious choices about what we eat can have a transformative effect on our overall health.

Inspiration from Barbara O'Neill

Drawing from Barbara's insights, this book is crafted to guide you gently but firmly on your weight loss journey. It's not about quick fixes or fleeting trends. Instead, it's about understanding your body, respecting its natural rhythms, and nurturing it with the right nutrients. Here, we will delve into the importance of whole foods, the role of different nutrients in weight management, and how to create meals that are not only nourishing but also delicious and satisfying.

As you turn these pages, remember that this journey is uniquely yours. Whether you're looking to shed a few pounds, overhaul your eating habits, or simply seek inspiration for healthier living, this book is your companion. Together, we will explore the art and science of eating well, all while keeping your individual needs and goals in mind.

So, let's begin this journey with an open heart and a willing spirit. Welcome to "Weight Loss Diet," where every meal is a step towards a healthier, happier you.

CHAPTER 1: UNDERSTANDING WEIGHT LOSS

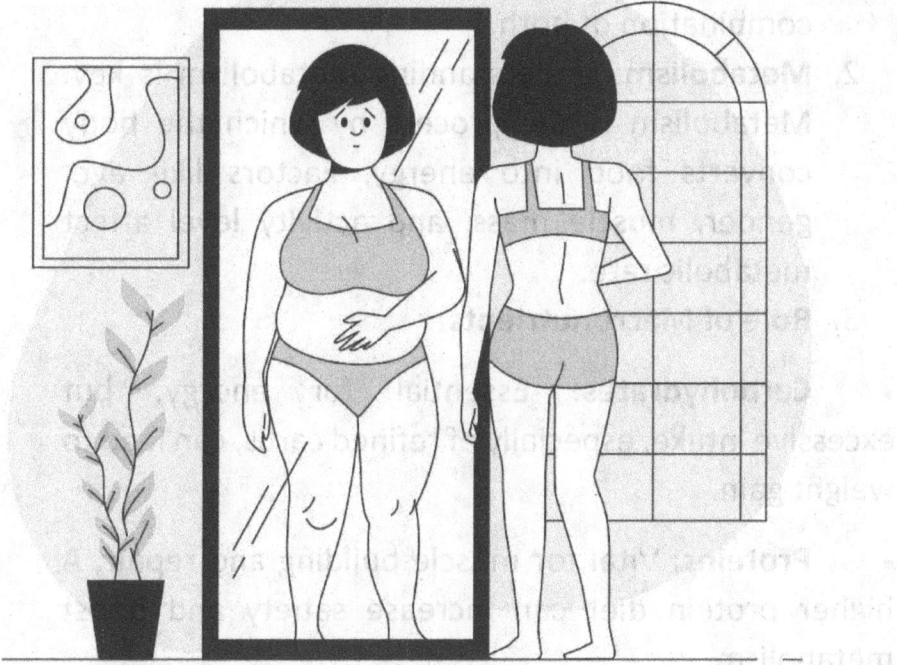

Understanding weight loss involves comprehending the underlying principles of how the body gains and loses weight, and implementing feasible strategies for achieving and maintaining a healthy weight. Let's explore this in depth.

1. **Caloric Balance**: Weight loss fundamentally comes down to the principle of caloric balance - consuming fewer calories than the body expends. This can be achieved through diet, exercise, or a combination of both.

2. **Metabolism**: Understanding metabolism is key. Metabolism is the process by which the body converts food into energy. Factors like age, gender, muscle mass, and activity level affect metabolic rate.

3. **Role of Macronutrients**:

• **Carbohydrates**: Essential for energy, but excessive intake, especially of refined carbs, can lead to weight gain.

• **Proteins**: Vital for muscle building and repair. A higher protein diet can increase satiety and boost metabolism.

• **Fats**: Necessary for hormonal function and nutrient absorption. Healthy fats are crucial, while trans and saturated fats should be limited.

Psychological Aspects

1. **Behavioral Change**: Sustainable weight loss often requires long-term behavioral changes in eating habits and physical activity.

2. **Emotional Eating**: Understanding the triggers for emotional eating and developing strategies to cope with stress can significantly impact weight management.
3. **Motivation and Mindset**: Maintaining a positive and realistic mindset is essential for long-term success.

Nutrition and Diet

1. **Whole Foods**: Emphasizing whole, unprocessed foods rich in nutrients can improve overall health and aid in weight loss.
2. **Portion Control**: Understanding and controlling portion sizes helps in maintaining a caloric deficit without the need for drastic diets.
3. **Balanced Meals**: A balance of macronutrients in each meal helps in sustaining energy levels and reducing cravings.

Physical Activity

1. **Exercise**: Regular physical activity increases caloric expenditure, helping create a caloric deficit. Both cardio and strength training are important.
2. **NEAT (Non-Exercise Activity Thermogenesis)**: Incorporating more movement into daily life, like

walking or taking the stairs, also contributes to weight loss.

Medical and Genetic Factors

1. **Health Conditions**: Certain health conditions and medications can impact weight. Consulting a healthcare provider can provide insights into any underlying issues.
2. **Genetics**: Genetics play a role in body weight, but they do not determine one's destiny. Lifestyle changes can still lead to significant improvements.

Making It Feasible

1. **Setting Realistic Goals**: Setting achievable short-term goals helps in staying motivated and tracking progress.
2. **Consistency Over Perfection**: Consistency in healthy eating and exercise is more effective than short-term, intense regimens.
3. **Support Systems**: Having a support system, whether it's friends, family, or a health professional, can greatly aid in the journey.
4. **Education and Resources**: Educating oneself about nutrition and health, possibly with the help of a dietician or similar professional, can provide the necessary tools and knowledge.
5. **Personalization**: Understanding that every individual is different, and customizing the approach to fit personal needs, preferences, and lifestyle.

In summary, understanding weight loss is about grasping the biological, psychological, and lifestyle factors that contribute to weight gain and loss. Implementing these principles in a practical, sustainable way is key to achieving long-term success in weight management.

The Basics of Metabolism

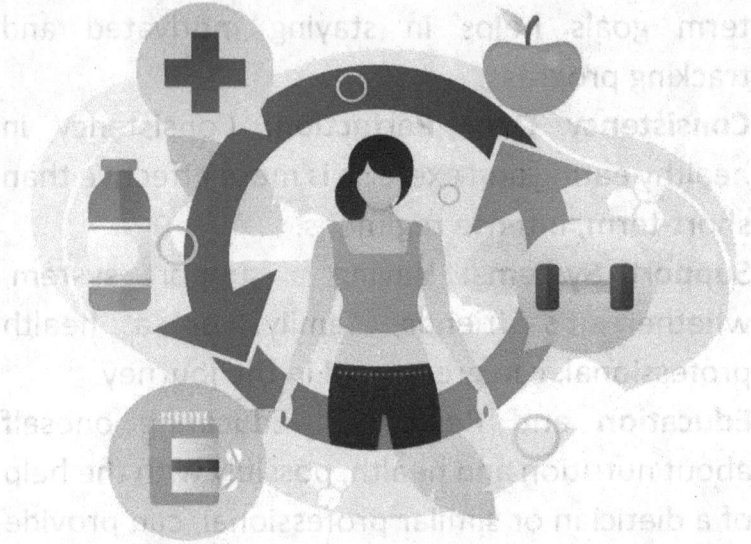

Metabolism refers to the complex biochemical processes that occur within a living organism to sustain life. It's primarily about how your body converts what you eat and drink into energy. This process is a balance of two activities: anabolism, which involves building and storing, and catabolism, the breakdown of molecules to produce energy.

The Role of Metabolism in Weight Management: Your metabolic rate influences how many calories you burn. A higher metabolism means you burn more calories at rest and during activity — a key player in weight loss and gain. However, it's a common misconception that a 'slow' metabolism leads to weight gain. In most cases, weight gain results from a complex interplay of genetic, hormonal, and lifestyle factors, with metabolism playing a smaller role.

Factors Affecting Metabolic Rate: Several factors influence your metabolic rate:

- **Age:** Metabolism naturally slows down as you age.

- **Muscle Mass:** More muscle mass equates to a higher metabolic rate.

- **Body Size:** Larger bodies may have a higher metabolic rate due to more energy requirements.

- **Gender:** Men often have less body fat and more muscle, slightly boosting their metabolism.

- **Physical Activity:** Regular exercise increases muscle mass and promotes a higher metabolic rate.

- **Hormonal Factors:** Thyroid problems and other hormonal imbalances can affect metabolism.

- **Environmental Factors:** Extreme cold or heat can increase metabolic rate as your body works to maintain normal temperature.

Metabolism and Caloric Intake: To lose weight, you must create a caloric deficit, burning more calories than you consume. Understanding your metabolic rate can guide your caloric intake needs. However, drastically reducing calories can be counterproductive, as it might slow down metabolism, making weight loss harder.

Boosting Your Metabolism: While genetics play a significant role, lifestyle changes can positively influence your metabolism:

• **Building Muscle:** Muscle is metabolically more active than fat. Strength training can help boost your metabolic rate.

• **Staying Active:** Regular physical activity, including aerobic exercises, can increase your metabolic rate.

• **Eating Protein-Rich Foods:** Protein-rich foods can temporarily boost metabolism more than fats or carbohydrates.

The Myth of 'Metabolism-Boosting' Products: Many products claim to boost metabolism, but there's limited scientific evidence to support these claims. Healthy lifestyle choices are a more effective and sustainable way to manage metabolism.

Understanding metabolism is essential in the context of diet and weight management. It's a complex process influenced by various factors, most of which are within your control through lifestyle choices. By focusing on building muscle, staying active, and eating a balanced diet, you can maintain a healthy metabolic rate conducive to achieving and maintaining a healthy weight.

Common Myths and Facts about Weight Loss

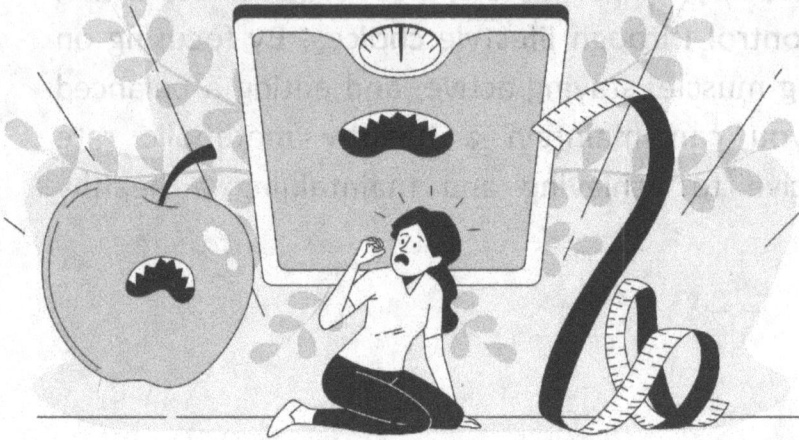

In a world bombarded with quick-fix diet plans and conflicting health advice, understanding the truth about weight loss is more critical than ever. Each day, new fads emerge, clouding our perception of what truly works. This section aims to dismantle 20 of the most prevalent myths surrounding weight loss, replacing them with facts grounded in scientific research. By doing so, we empower ourselves to make informed decisions that lead to healthier, sustainable lifestyle changes.

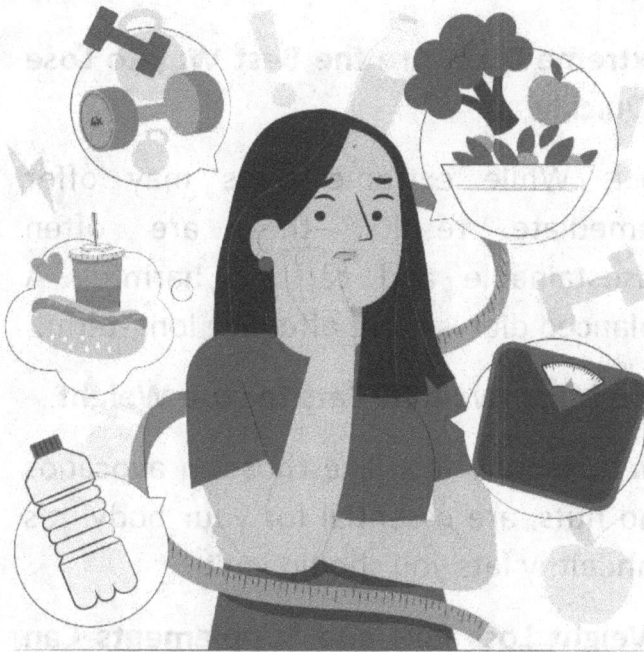

1. **Myth: Skipping Meals Promotes Faster Weight Loss**

    - *Fact*: Skipping meals can slow down your metabolism and lead to overeating later. Regular, balanced meals are key to a healthy metabolism.

2. **Myth: All Calories Are Created Equal**

    - *Fact*: The type of calories matters. Calories from whole foods like fruits and vegetables are far more beneficial than calories from processed foods.

3. **Myth: Extreme Diets Are the Best Way to Lose Weight Quickly**

   - *Fact*: While extreme diets may offer immediate results, they are often unsustainable and can be harmful. A balanced diet is more effective long-term.

4. **Myth: You Must Avoid All Fats to Lose Weight**

   - *Fact*: Healthy fats, like those in avocados and nuts, are essential for your body. It's unhealthy fats you should limit.

5. **Myth: Weight Loss Pills and Supplements Can Replace Diet and Exercise**

   - *Fact*: There's no magic pill for weight loss. Sustainable weight loss requires a combination of dietary changes and physical activity.

6. **Myth: "Diet" Foods Are Always a Healthy Choice**

   - *Fact*: Foods labeled as "diet" or "low-fat" can be misleading and may contain high levels of sugar and artificial ingredients.

7. **Myth: Carbohydrates Make You Gain Weight**

- *Fact*: While refined carbs should be limited, whole grains, fruits, and vegetables are healthy and necessary for energy.

8. **Myth: Eating Late at Night Causes Weight Gain**

   - *Fact*: It's not when you eat, but what and how much you eat. Overeating, regardless of the time, leads to weight gain.

9. **Myth: You Should Weigh Yourself Every Day**

   - *Fact*: Daily weight fluctuations are normal. It's more helpful to track your weight over longer periods.

10. **Myth: Exercise Alone Can Lead to Weight Loss**

    - *Fact*: While exercise is crucial, diet plays a more significant role in weight loss. Both are essential for overall health.

11. **Myth: High-Intensity Exercise is the Only Way to Lose Weight**

    - *Fact*: A mix of moderate and high-intensity exercise can be effective. Consistency is more important than intensity.

12. **Myth: Gluten-Free Diets Aid in Weight Loss**

- *Fact*: Gluten-free diets are essential for those with celiac disease, but they don't inherently lead to weight loss.

13. **Myth: Drinking Water Before Meals Reduces Hunger**

    - *Fact*: While staying hydrated is important, water alone does not significantly affect hunger levels.

14. **Myth: You Need to Cut Out All Sugar to Lose Weight**

    - *Fact*: While reducing added sugars is beneficial, eliminating all sugar, including natural sugars in fruits, isn't necessary.

15. **Myth: Vegetarian or Vegan Diets Automatically Lead to Weight Loss**

    - *Fact*: Plant-based diets can be healthy, but weight loss still depends on overall calorie intake and food choices.

16. **Myth: You Can Target Fat Loss in Specific Areas**

    - *Fact*: Spot reduction is a myth. Fat loss occurs throughout the body based on genetics and overall body fat percentage.

17.**Myth: Eating Small, Frequent Meals Boosts Metabolism**

- *Fact*: Metabolic rate is more dependent on total food intake and composition rather than meal frequency.

18.**Myth: Low-Intensity Exercises Like Walking Aren't Effective for Weight Loss**

- *Fact*: Low-intensity exercises, especially when consistent, can contribute significantly to weight loss and overall health.

19.**Myth: You Shouldn't Eat Before a Workout**

- *Fact*: A light snack before exercise can provide energy. The key is what and how much you eat.

20.**Myth: Losing Weight is a Linear Process**

- *Fact*: Weight loss often involves plateaus and fluctuations. It's a journey with ups and downs, not a straight line.

21.**Myth: You Should Only Focus on Cardio for Weight Loss**

- *Fact*: Strength training is equally important as it builds muscle, which can increase metabolism and aid in weight loss.

22. **Myth: Fat-Free Foods are Always Better for Losing Weight**

    - *Fact*: Many fat-free products compensate by adding sugar or other unhealthy ingredients. Balance is key.

23. **Myth: You Can Lose Weight Without Changing Your Diet If You Exercise Enough**

    - *Fact*: Diet plays a crucial role in weight loss. Exercise alone is usually not enough without dietary changes.

24. **Myth: You Shouldn't Eat After 6 PM to Lose Weight**

    - *Fact*: It's the total calorie intake and expenditure over the day that matters, not the time you eat.

25. **Myth: You Have to Give Up Your Favorite Foods to Lose Weight**

    - *Fact*: Moderation and portion control are essential. You can enjoy your favorite foods in smaller amounts.

26. **Myth: Certain Foods Like Grapefruit or Cabbage Burn Fat**

   - *Fact*: No food can burn fat. These diets are fads and not supported by scientific evidence.

27. **Myth: You Can Sweat Out Fat**

   - *Fact*: Sweat is not fat leaving the body; it's the body regulating its temperature.

28. **Myth: Eating Protein Alone Leads to Weight Loss**

   - *Fact*: While protein is essential for muscle building and satiety, a balanced diet is crucial for healthy weight loss.

29. **Myth: Juicing or Detox Diets Are Effective and Sustainable Weight Loss Strategies**

   - *Fact*: These diets can lead to temporary weight loss but are often not sustainable and lack essential nutrients.

30. **Myth: More Gym Time Always Equals More Weight Loss**

   - *Fact*: Quality and intensity of exercise can be more important than duration. Overtraining can also be counterproductive.

31. **Myth: If You're Not Losing Weight, You're Not Making Progress**

   - *Fact*: Muscle weighs more than fat. You can be getting healthier and more toned even if the scale doesn't change.

32. **Myth: Eating at Night Makes You Fat**

   - *Fact*: It's the total calorie intake, not the time of consumption, that influences weight gain.

33. **Myth: Fasting Jumpstarts Weight Loss**

   - *Fact*: While fasting can reduce weight initially, it can also slow metabolism and lead to muscle loss.

34. **Myth: Thin Equals Healthy**

   - *Fact*: Health is not solely determined by weight. Thin people can have health issues, and overweight people can be healthy.

35. **Myth: You Can Trust All Weight Loss Advice on Social Media**

   - *Fact*: Always seek advice from qualified professionals. Social media can be full of unverified and potentially harmful tips.

36. **Myth: It's Possible to Get Abs Just by Doing Crunches**

- *Fact*: Abs are made in the kitchen and the gym. Diet and overall body fat reduction are key.

37. **Myth: Cutting Out Dairy Helps You Lose Weight**

- *Fact*: Unless you're lactose intolerant, dairy is a good source of calcium and protein and doesn't need to be eliminated.

38. **Myth: Weight Loss is a Quick Process**

- *Fact*: Sustainable weight loss is often slow. Quick weight loss methods are usually unhealthy or temporary.

39. **Myth: Salads Are Always the Best Diet Food**

- *Fact*: Salads can be healthy, but toppings and dressings can add excess calories. Ingredients matter.

40. **Myth: Weight Loss Supplements Don't Have Side Effects**

- *Fact*: Many supplements can have harmful side effects and are not regulated as strictly as medications.

41. **Myth: You Can Compensate for a Bad Diet with Exercise**

- *Fact*: Diet plays a critical role in weight management. Exercise cannot fully compensate for poor dietary habits.

42. **Myth: Brown Sugar is Healthier than White Sugar for Weight Loss**

- *Fact*: Brown sugar is slightly less refined but has a similar calorie content as white sugar.

43. **Myth: You Must Reach a Certain Weight to Be Healthy**

- *Fact*: Health is multifaceted. It's more about body composition, fitness, and overall wellbeing than just weight.

44. **Myth: Bigger Portions of Healthy Food Won't Affect Weight**

- *Fact*: Even with healthy foods, calorie intake matters. Portion control is essential.

45. **Myth: You Should Aim for the 'Ideal Weight' on Charts**

- *Fact*: Ideal weight charts don't consider body composition and individual differences. Focus on healthy body composition.

46. **Myth: All Smoothies and Protein Shakes Are Good for Weight Loss**

   - *Fact*: Some can be high in sugar and calories. It's important to know the ingredients.

47. **Myth: Weight Loss is Just About Willpower**

   - *Fact*: It's more complex involving psychological, physiological, and environmental factors.

48. **Myth: Certain Exercises Can Slim Down Your Hips and Thighs**

   - *Fact*: You cannot target where you lose fat. Body shape is influenced by genetics and overall fat loss.

49. **Myth: "Cheat Days" Are Necessary for a Successful Diet**

   - *Fact*: While occasional indulgences are okay, terming them as "cheat days" can promote an unhealthy relationship with food.

50. **Myth: You Can't Eat Any Sweets or Treats When on a Diet**

- *Fact*: Deprivation isn't sustainable. Small treats, in moderation, can be part of a healthy diet.

In conclusion, understanding these myths and their realities is vital in navigating the complex world of weight loss. By embracing a balanced approach to diet and exercise, informed by facts rather than fads, you're more likely to achieve sustainable results and improved overall health.

CHAPTER 2: PRINCIPLES OF A HEALTHY DIET

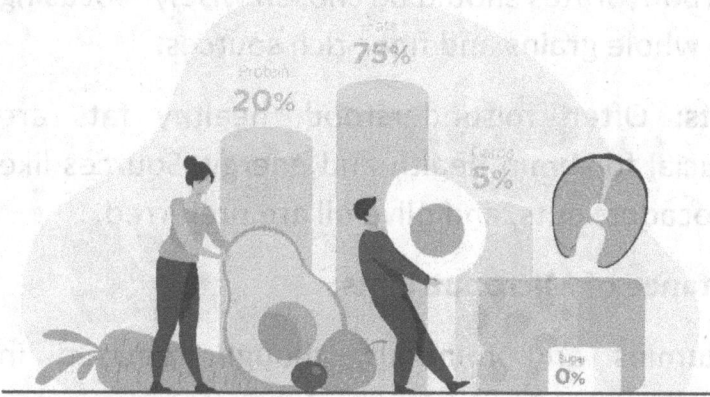

Setting out on a journey towards a healthier lifestyle begins with understanding the core principles of a healthy diet. This chapter delves into the fundamentals of nutrition and extracts valuable lessons from Barbara O'Neill's "Self Heal by Design." We aim to build a bridge between the foundational knowledge of what constitutes a nutritious diet and the practical wisdom shared by O'Neill, creating a holistic approach to weight loss and overall health.

Nutrition Fundamentals

1. Macronutrients and Their Roles:

- **Proteins:** Essential for muscle repair and growth, proteins are the building blocks of our body.

- **Carbohydrates:** The primary source of energy, carbohydrates should be chosen wisely - focusing on whole grains and fiber-rich sources.

- **Fats:** Often misunderstood, healthy fats are crucial for brain health and energy. Sources like avocados, nuts, and olive oil are preferred.

2. Importance of Micronutrients:

- Vitamins and minerals, though required in smaller quantities, play vital roles in various bodily functions, from immune response to bone health.

3. Hydration:

- Water is central to life. It aids in digestion, nutrient absorption, and detoxification.

4. Understanding Calories:

- A balance between calorie intake and expenditure is key to weight management. It's not just about quantity but also the quality of calories.

Lessons from 'Self Heal by Design'

Barbara O'Neill emphasizes the power of natural healing through diet. Let's draw key lessons from her work:

1. The Power of Whole Foods:

- O'Neill advocates for a diet rich in whole, unprocessed foods. These foods are closer to their natural state and retain more nutrients.

2. The Role of Plant-Based Foods:

- A significant emphasis is placed on plant-based diets - rich in fruits, vegetables, and whole grains, which are not only nutrient-dense but also high in fiber.

3. Listening to Your Body:

- O'Neill suggests tuning into your body's signals. Understanding hunger cues and eating mindfully plays a crucial role in a healthy diet.

4. The Detoxification Principle:

- The importance of regular detoxification through diet is highlighted. Foods that naturally cleanse the body, like leafy greens and citrus fruits, are encouraged.

5. The Holistic Approach:

- O'Neill's approach is not just about what we eat but how we eat. Stress management, adequate sleep, and emotional well-being are integral.

Understanding these principles is just the first step. The real magic happens when we synergize this knowledge with practical application. In the upcoming chapters, we'll see how these principles are not just theories but tools for crafting a lifestyle that embraces wholesome nutrition and mindful eating, leading to sustainable weight loss and enhanced well-being.

As we move forward, keep in mind that a healthy diet is not a one-size-fits-all solution; it's a personal journey that respects your body's unique needs and preferences, aligning with the wisdom shared by Barbara O'Neill in "Self Heal by Design."

CHAPTER 3: PREPARING FOR YOUR WEIGHT LOSS JOURNEY

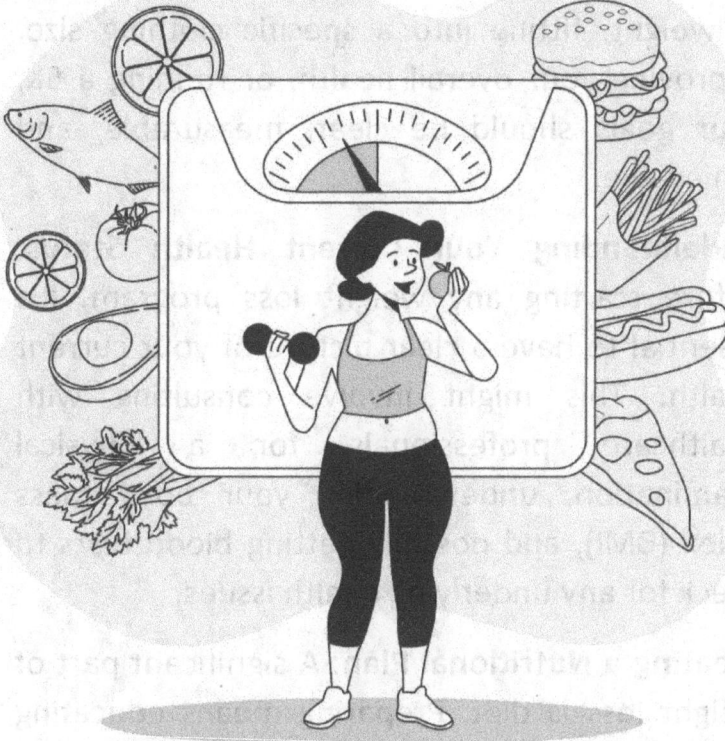

Preparing for a weight loss journey involves several key steps, each designed to set you up for success in achieving your health and fitness goals. It's a holistic approach that encompasses physical, mental, and logistical preparations:

1. **Setting Realistic Goals**: This is about understanding what you want to achieve and setting targets that are attainable and sustainable. Whether it's losing a certain amount of weight, fitting into a specific clothing size, improving your overall health, or running a 5K, your goals should be clear, measurable, and achievable.

2. **Understanding Your Current Health Status**: Before starting any weight loss program, it's essential to have a clear picture of your current health. This might involve consulting with healthcare professionals for a physical examination, understanding your body mass index (BMI), and possibly getting blood tests to check for any underlying health issues.

3. **Creating a Nutritional Plan**: A significant part of weight loss is diet. Preparing means educating yourself about nutrition, perhaps with the help of a dietitian or nutritionist. It involves planning meals that are balanced, portion-controlled, and in line with your weight loss goals.

4. **Establishing an Exercise Routine**: Exercise is a crucial component of weight loss. Preparing for your journey may involve finding a type of exercise you enjoy, setting a consistent workout

schedule, and possibly consulting with a fitness trainer.

5. **Mental and Emotional Preparation**: Weight loss is not just a physical challenge; it's a mental and emotional one as well. Preparing yourself mentally involves cultivating a positive mindset, setting realistic expectations, and developing strategies to handle potential setbacks and challenges.

6. **Organizing Your Environment**: This includes setting up your living space to support your weight loss goals. It might mean stocking your kitchen with healthy foods, getting rid of tempting unhealthy snacks, and creating a dedicated space for exercise.

7. **Building a Support System**: Having a network of support can greatly enhance your weight loss journey. This could be friends, family, a weight loss group, or an online community. People who understand your goals and can offer encouragement and accountability are invaluable.

8. **Planning for Obstacles**: Anticipating and planning for potential obstacles, like busy schedules, holidays, or emotional triggers, can help you stay

on track. This might involve learning strategies for healthy eating during travel, managing stress without turning to food or finding ways to stay active even during busy times.

Preparing for a weight loss journey is about laying a foundation for a healthier lifestyle. It's a process that requires thought, planning, and commitment, but with the right preparation, your journey can be more effective, enjoyable, and sustainable.

The Art of Setting Realistic Goals

Setting realistic goals is the cornerstone of this endeavor, ensuring that each step taken is a step closer to overall health and wellbeing. Below are some factors to note while setting out realistic weight loss goals;

1. **Understanding Personal Limitations and Strengths**

   - Every journey begins with self-awareness. Understanding your body, your dietary preferences, and your lifestyle is crucial. It's not just about shedding pounds; it's about embracing a healthier lifestyle that fits seamlessly into your daily routine.

2. **SMART Goals: Specific, Measurable, Achievable, Relevant, Time-Bound**

- A goal without a plan is just a wish. SMART goals provide a framework for setting objectives that are clear, attainable, and time-sensitive. For example, aiming to lose 1-2 pounds per week is more practical than a vague goal of "losing weight."

3. **The Role of Incremental Changes**

- Rome wasn't built in a day, and similarly, lasting weight loss doesn't happen overnight. Small, incremental changes in diet and lifestyle are more sustainable than drastic overhauls. This could mean starting by cutting out sugary drinks before overhauling your entire diet.

4. **Balancing Aspirations with Patience**

- Weight loss is a journey of ebbs and flows. It requires patience and understanding that progress might be slow and non-linear. Celebrating small victories along the way keeps motivation high and reinforces the positive impact of the changes you're making.

5. **Customizing Goals to Fit Individual Lifestyles**

- What works for one may not work for another. Tailoring goals to fit individual schedules, dietary preferences, and exercise capabilities is essential. This personalization makes the journey more enjoyable and the goals more attainable.

6. **Seeking Professional Guidance When Needed**

   - Consulting with dietitians, nutritionists, or personal trainers can provide valuable insights into setting realistic goals. These professionals can offer tailored advice based on your health history and personal objectives.

7. **The Importance of Flexibility**

   - Life is unpredictable, and rigid goals can become a source of frustration. Flexibility allows for adjustments in response to life's changes, ensuring that your weight loss journey remains a positive and adaptive part of your life.

Setting realistic goals is not just about reducing numbers on a scale; it's about embarking on a journey towards a healthier, more fulfilling life. By understanding personal needs, setting SMART goals, embracing incremental changes, and staying flexible, the path to weight loss becomes not only achievable but also enjoyable. Remember, the journey of a thousand miles begins with a single, well-planned step.

Essential Kitchen Tools and Ingredients that aids weight loss

The adage "You are what you eat" is a cornerstone of health, and in this chapter, we will delve into the essential kitchen tools and ingredients that aid in weight loss, ensuring your culinary space is not just a kitchen, but a haven for healthful living.

Essential Kitchen Tools for Weight Loss

1. **Digital Food Scale:** Precision is key in portion control.

2. **Measuring Cups and Spoons:** For accurate ingredient measurements.

3. **Blender:** Ideal for smoothies and purees.

4. **Food Processor:** To quickly chop and blend ingredients.

5. **Non-Stick Skillet:** Reduces the need for excess oil.

6. **Air Fryer:** For healthier frying options.

7. **Steamer Basket:** Preserves nutrients in vegetables.

8. **Slow Cooker:** For easy, healthy meals.

9. **Pressure Cooker:** Speeds up cooking time.

10. **Salad Spinner:** For clean, crisp greens.

11. **Oil Mister:** Controls the amount of oil used.

12. **Vegetable Spiralizer:** For creating veggie noodles.

13. **Mandoline Slicer:** For uniform vegetable slices.

14. **Garlic Press:** Effortless garlic mincing.

15. **Citrus Juicer:** For fresh juice without added sugars.

16. **Herb Scissors:** For easily chopping fresh herbs.

17. **Spice Grinder:** To freshly grind spices.

18. **Kitchen Thermometer:** Ensures proper cooking temperatures.

19. **Grill Pan:** For indoor grilling.

20. **Mixing Bowls:** Various sizes for meal prep.

21. **Baking Sheets:** For roasting vegetables and meats.

22. **Glass Storage Containers:** For meal prep and storage.

23. **Salad Dressing Shaker:** For homemade dressings.

24. **Fine Mesh Strainer:** For rinsing grains and legumes.

25. **Peeler:** Essential for prepping fruits and veggies.

26. **Chopping Knives:** A good set for all purposes.

27. **Cutting Boards:** Preferably in multiple sizes.

28. **Spatulas and Turners:** For flipping and stirring.

29. **Ladle and Serving Spoons:** For soups and stews.

30. **Can Opener:** For canned beans, tomatoes, etc.

31. **Colander:** For draining pasta and washing veggies.

32. **Microplane Grater:** For zesting and fine grating.

33. **Silicone Baking Mats:** For non-stick baking.

34. **Oven Mitts:** To handle hot dishes safely.

35. **Kitchen Timer:** To keep track of cooking times.

36. **Vegetable Brush:** To thoroughly clean produce.

37. **Immersion Blender:** For blending soups and sauces.

38. **Rolling Pin:** For healthy homemade dough.

39. **Bread Knife:** For slicing whole grain bread.

40. **Tea Infuser:** For brewing herbal teas.

41. **Egg Poacher:** For healthy egg preparation.

42. **Rice Cooker:** For perfect grains every time.

43. **Coffee Grinder:** Freshly ground coffee beans.

44. **Milk Frother:** For healthy coffee additions.

45. **Digital Kitchen Timer:** For precise cooking times.

46. **Pastry Brush:** For minimal oil brushing.

47. **Cheese Grater:** For controlled cheese portions.

48. **Meat Tenderizer:** For lean meats.

49. **Pasta Maker:** For homemade, healthy pasta.

50. **Ice Cream Maker:** For healthy frozen treats.

Some Essential Ingredients for Weight Loss

51. **Quinoa:** A high-protein, versatile grain.

52. **Brown Rice:** A whole grain, fiber-rich option.

53. **Oats:** For heart-healthy breakfasts.

54. **Almonds:** A good source of healthy fats.

55. **Walnuts:** Rich in omega-3 fatty acids.

56. **Chia Seeds:** High in fiber and omega-3s.

57. **Flaxseeds:** Great for adding to smoothies and yogurts.

58. **Lentils:** A great source of plant-based protein.

59. **Chickpeas:** Versatile and high in protein.

60. **Black Beans:** Fiber-rich and filling.

61. **Tofu:** A low-calorie, high-protein option.

62. **Greek Yogurt:** High in protein and probiotics.

63. **Skim Milk:** A low-fat dairy choice.

64. **Spinach:** Rich in vitamins and low in calories.

65. **Kale:** A nutrient-dense leafy green.

66. **Broccoli:** High in fiber and vitamins.

67. **Bell Peppers:** Low in calories, high in flavor.

68. **Sweet Potatoes:** A healthier carb option.

69. **Avocado:** Healthy fats for satiety.

70. **Berries:** Low in calories, high in antioxidants.

71. **Apples:** A fiber-rich snack.

72. **Bananas:** Potassium-rich and filling.

73. **Whole Grain Bread:** A better choice than white bread.

74. **Eggs:** A versatile protein source.

75. **Chicken Breast:** Lean protein.

76. **Salmon:** Rich in omega-3 fatty acids.

77. **Turkey:** A lean meat option.

78. **Garlic:** Adds flavor without calories.

79. **Onions:** A base for many healthy dishes.

80. **Tomatoes:** Low in calories, high in vitamins.

81. **Cucumbers:** Hydrating and low in calories.

82. **Zucchini:** Versatile and low in carbs.

83. **Carrots:** Good for snacking and rich in beta-carotene.

84. **Lemons/Limes:** For flavor without extra calories.

85. **Vinegar (like apple cider):** For dressings and marinades.

86. **Herbs (like basil, and cilantro):** For flavor without fat.

87. **Spices (like turmeric, and cinnamon):** Metabolism boosters.

88. **Green Tea:** Aids in metabolism.

89. **Dark Chocolate:** For a healthy treat in moderation.

90. **Whole Wheat Pasta:** A better pasta option.

91. **Almond Milk:** A low-calorie dairy alternative.

92. **Coconut Oil:** A healthier cooking oil option.

93. **Olive Oil:** Ideal for heart-healthy cooking.

94. **Honey:** A natural sweetener.

95. **Maple Syrup:** Another natural sweetener.

96. **Dijon Mustard:** For flavor in dressings and marinades.

97. **Low-Sodium Soy Sauce:** For flavor without the bloat.

98. **Canned Tomatoes:** A pantry staple for healthy sauces.

99. **Frozen Vegetables:** Convenient and nutritious.

100. **Frozen Berries:** For smoothies and desserts.

In the next chapter, we will explore how to utilize these tools and ingredients to craft delicious, healthy recipes that aid in weight loss, ensuring a seamless transition from theory to practice in your culinary journey.

CHAPTER 4: WEIGHT LOSS DIET RECIPES

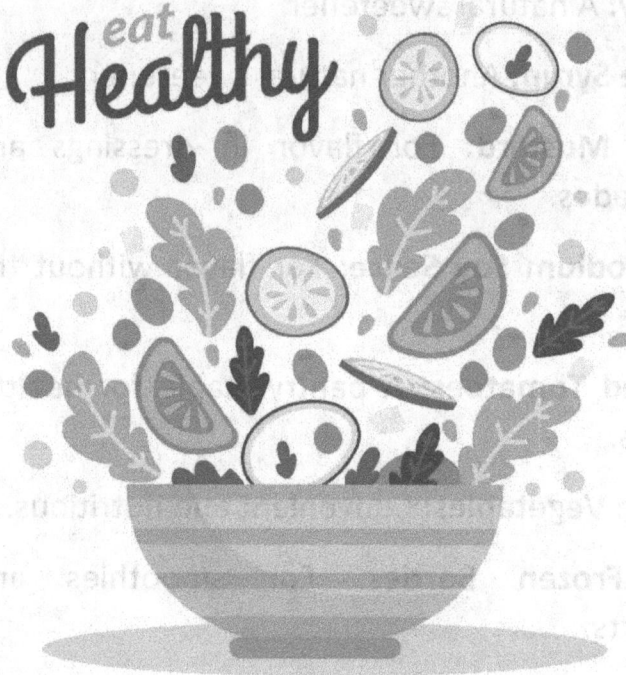

Here are 10 nutritious breakfast recipes tailored for a weight loss diet. Each recipe is designed to be both delicious and health-conscious, helping to kickstart your metabolism while keeping you satisfied.

10 Nutritious Breakfast Recipes

1. Berry and Spinach Breakfast Smoothie Bowl

Preparation Time: 10 Minutes | Total Time: 15 Minutes | Makes 2 Servings

Ingredients:

- 1 cup mixed berries (frozen or fresh – such as strawberries, blueberries, raspberries)
- 1 ripe banana
- 1 cup fresh spinach leaves
- 1/2 cup Greek yogurt, low-fat
- 1/4 cup almond milk
- 2 tablespoons rolled oats
- 1 tablespoon honey (optional)
- Toppings: Sliced almonds, chia seeds, additional berries, and a sprinkle of granola

Directions:

- In a blender, combine the mixed berries, banana, spinach, Greek yogurt, almond milk, rolled oats, and honey (if using). Blend until smooth and creamy.
- If the mixture is too thick, add a little more almond milk to reach the desired consistency.

- Pour the smoothie mixture into two bowls.
- Garnish each bowl with sliced almonds, chia seeds, additional berries, and a sprinkle of granola for added texture and nutrients.
- Serve immediately for a fresh, energizing start to your day.

Nutrition per serving: Calories 220 | Total Fat 4g | Sat Fat 1g | Carbs 40g | Fiber 7g | Protein 10g | Sodium 55mg

2. Avocado Toast with Poached Egg

Preparation Time: 10 Minutes | Total Time: 15 Minutes | Makes 1 Serving

Ingredients:

- 1 slice whole grain bread
- 1/2 ripe avocado, mashed
- 1 egg, poached
- Pinch of red pepper flakes
- Salt and pepper to taste

Directions:

- Toast the bread to your liking.
- Spread the mashed avocado on the toast.
- Place the poached egg on top.
- Season with red pepper flakes, salt, and pepper.

Nutrition per serving: Calories 250 | Total Fat 15g | Sat Fat 3g | Carbs 20g | Fiber 7g | Protein 10g | Sodium 210mg

3. Oatmeal with Almond Butter and Banana

Preparation Time: 5 Minutes | Cooking Time: 5 Minutes | Makes 1 Serving

Ingredients:

- 1/2 cup rolled oats
- 1 cup water or almond milk
- 1 tablespoon almond butter
- 1 banana, sliced

Directions:

- Cook the oats in water or almond milk according to package instructions.
- Stir in the almond butter.
- Top with sliced banana.

Nutrition per serving: Calories 330 | Total Fat 10g | Sat Fat 1g | Carbs 53g | Fiber 8g | Protein 11g | Sodium 10mg

4. Spinach and Mushroom Omelette

Preparation Time: 5 Minutes | Cooking Time: 10 Minutes | Makes 1 Serving

Ingredients:

- 2 eggs
- 1 cup fresh spinach, chopped
- 1/2 cup mushrooms, sliced
- Salt and pepper to taste
- Cooking spray

Directions:

- Beat the eggs in a bowl.
- Spray a pan with cooking spray and cook the spinach and mushrooms until soft.
- Pour the eggs over the vegetables. Cook until the eggs are set.
- Fold the omelet and serve.

Nutrition per serving: Calories 180 | Total Fat 10g | Sat Fat 3g | Carbs 5g | Fiber 2g | Protein 16g | Sodium 200mg

5. Chia Seed Pudding with Coconut and Mango

Preparation Time: 10 Minutes (plus overnight soaking) | Total Time: 10 Minutes | Makes 1 Serving

Ingredients:

- 3 tablespoons chia seeds
- 3/4 cup coconut milk (light)
- 1/2 mango, diced
- 1 tablespoon shredded coconut

Directions:

- Mix the chia seeds and coconut milk in a bowl. Refrigerate overnight.
- Top with diced mango and shredded coconut before serving.

Nutrition per serving: Calories 300 | Total Fat 18g | Sat Fat 8g | Carbs 35g | Fiber 10g | Protein 6g | Sodium 15mg

6. Smoked Salmon and Avocado Wrap

Preparation Time: 10 Minutes | Total Time: 10 Minutes | Makes 1 Serving

Ingredients:

- 1 whole grain wrap
- 2 oz smoked salmon
- 1/4 avocado, sliced
- 1 tablespoon cream cheese, low-fat
- Spinach leaves
- Sliced cucumber

Directions:

- Spread the cream cheese on the wrap.
- Add the smoked salmon, avocado, spinach, and cucumber.
- Roll up the wrap and cut it in half.

Nutrition per serving: Calories 320 | Total Fat 15g | Sat Fat 4g | Carbs 28g | Fiber 6g | Protein 20g | Sodium 560mg

7. Cottage Cheese and Pineapple Bowl
Preparation Time: 5 Minutes | Total Time: 5 Minutes | Makes 1 Serving

Ingredients:

- 1/2 cup cottage cheese, low-fat
- 1/2 cup pineapple, chopped
- 1 tablespoon almonds, sliced

Directions:

- Mix the cottage cheese with the pineapple.
- Top with sliced almonds.

Nutrition per serving: Calories 180 | Total Fat 5g | Sat Fat 1g | Carbs 20g | Fiber 2g | Protein 15g | Sodium 350mg

8. Veggie Breakfast Burrito Preparation Time: 10 Minutes | Cooking Time: 10 Minutes | Makes 1 Serving

Ingredients:

- 1 whole grain tortilla
- 2 egg whites
- 1/4 cup bell peppers, diced
- 1/4 cup onions, diced
- 1/4 cup black beans, rinsed and drained
- 1 tablespoon salsa
- 1 tablespoon shredded cheese, low-fat

Directions:

- Cook the egg whites in a pan until set.
- Add the bell peppers and onions, and cook until soft.
- Warm the tortilla, then place the egg mixture, black beans, salsa, and cheese in the center.
- Roll up the burrito.

Nutrition per serving: Calories 250 | Total Fat 6g | Sat Fat 2g | Carbs 35g | Fiber 8g | Protein 18g | Sodium 500mg

9. Blueberry Almond Overnight Oats

Preparation Time: 5 Minutes (plus overnight soaking) | Total Time: 5 Minutes | Makes 1 Serving

Ingredients:

- 1/2 cup rolled oats
- 1/2 cup almond milk
- 1/4 cup blueberries
- 1 tablespoon almond butter
- 1 teaspoon honey (optional)

Directions:

- Combine oats, almond milk, blueberries, and almond butter in a jar.
- Refrigerate overnight.
- Top with honey before serving (if desired).

Nutrition per serving: Calories 310 | Total Fat 12g | Sat Fat 1g | Carbs 45g | Fiber 7g | Protein 10g | Sodium 80mg

10.   Turkey and Spinach Scramble Preparation Time: 5 Minutes | Cooking Time: 10 Minutes | Makes 1 Serving

Ingredients:

- 3 egg whites
- 2 oz turkey breast, chopped
- 1 cup spinach, chopped
- Salt and pepper to taste
- Cooking spray

Directions:

- Spray a pan with cooking spray. Cook the turkey breast until browned.
- Add the spinach and cook until wilted.
- Add the egg whites and scramble together. Season with salt and pepper.

Nutrition per serving: Calories 160 | Total Fat 2g | Sat Fat 0g | Carbs 3g | Fiber 1g | Protein 28g | Sodium 400mg

10 Healthy Lunch Recipes

1. Chickpea and Quinoa Salad Bowl

Preparation Time: 20 Minutes | Total Time: 40 Minutes | Makes 6 Servings

Ingredients:

- 1 cup quinoa, rinsed
- 2 cups water
- 1 can (15 ounces) chickpeas, drained and rinsed
- 1 cucumber, diced
- 1 red bell pepper, diced
- 1/2 red onion, finely chopped
- 1/4 cup fresh parsley, chopped
- 1/4 cup olive oil
- Juice of 1 lemon
- 1 garlic clove, minced
- 1/2 teaspoon ground cumin
- Salt and pepper, to taste

Directions:

1. In a medium saucepan, bring the 2 cups of water to a boil. Add quinoa, reduce heat to low,

cover, and simmer for about 15 minutes, or until all water is absorbed. Remove from heat and let stand for 5 minutes, then fluff with a fork.

2. In a large bowl, combine cooked quinoa, chickpeas, cucumber, red bell pepper, red onion, and parsley.

3. In a small bowl, whisk together olive oil, lemon juice, minced garlic, cumin, salt, and pepper to create the dressing.

4. Pour the dressing over the quinoa mixture and toss gently to combine.

5. Serve immediately, or refrigerate to let flavors blend.

Nutrition per serving: Calories: 220 | Total Fat: 8g | Sat Fat: 1g | Carbs: 31g | Fiber: 6g | Protein: 8g | Sodium: 15mg

2. Spinach and Strawberry Salad with Grilled Chicken

Preparation Time: 15 Minutes | Total Time: 30 Minutes | Makes 4 Servings

Ingredients:

- 4 boneless, skinless chicken breasts
- 8 cups fresh spinach leaves
- 1 cup strawberries, sliced
- 1/4 cup sliced almonds
- 1/4 cup crumbled feta cheese
- 2 tablespoons balsamic vinegar
- 1 tablespoon olive oil
- Salt and pepper to taste

Directions:

1. Season chicken breasts with salt and pepper. Grill over medium heat until cooked through, about 6-7 minutes per side.

2. In a large bowl, combine spinach, strawberries, almonds, and feta cheese.

3. Slice grilled chicken and add to the salad.

4. Drizzle with balsamic vinegar and olive oil, toss gently, and serve.

Nutrition per serving: Calories: 250 | Total Fat: 9g | Sat Fat: 2g | Carbs: 10g | Fiber: 3g | Protein: 35g | Sodium: 200mg

3. Mediterranean Tuna Salad

4. Preparation Time: 15 Minutes | Makes 4 Servings

Ingredients:

- 2 cans (5 ounces each) of tuna in water, drained
- 1/2 cup cherry tomatoes, halved
- 1/4 cup red onion, finely chopped
- 1/4 cup Kalamata olives, pitted and chopped
- 1/4 cup feta cheese, crumbled
- 2 tablespoons olive oil
- 1 tablespoon lemon juice
- Salt and pepper to taste
- 4 cups mixed salad greens

Directions:

1. In a bowl, mix tuna, tomatoes, red onion, olives, and feta cheese.

2. In a small bowl, whisk together olive oil, lemon juice, salt, and pepper.

3. Pour dressing over tuna mixture and toss gently.

4. Serve over a bed of mixed salad greens.

Nutrition per serving: Calories: 180 | Total Fat: 10g | Sat Fat: 2g | Carbs: 4g | Fiber: 1g | Protein: 20g | Sodium: 320mg

5. Asian-Inspired Turkey Lettuce Wraps

Preparation Time: 15 Minutes | Cook Time: 10 Minutes | Makes 4 Servings

Ingredients:

- 1 pound ground turkey
- 1 tablespoon sesame oil
- 2 cloves garlic, minced
- 1 tablespoon ginger, grated
- 1/4 cup hoisin sauce
- 2 green onions, chopped
- 1 head iceberg lettuce, leaves separated

Directions:

1. Heat sesame oil in a skillet over medium heat. Add garlic and ginger, and sauté for 1 minute.

2. Add ground turkey and cook until browned.

3. Stir in hoisin sauce and green onions, and cook for another 2 minutes.

4. Serve the turkey mixture in lettuce leaves.

Nutrition per serving: Calories: 220 | Total Fat: 10g | Sat Fat: 2g | Carbs: 12g | Fiber: 1g | Protein: 23g | Sodium: 500mg

5. Quinoa and Black Bean Stuffed Peppers
Preparation Time: 20 Minutes | Cook Time: 25 Minutes | Makes 4 Servings

Ingredients:

- 4 bell peppers, tops cut off and seeds removed
- 1 cup cooked quinoa
- 1 can (15 ounces) black beans, drained and rinsed
- 1/2 cup corn kernels
- 1/2 cup tomato, chopped
- 1/4 cup cilantro, chopped
- 1/2 teaspoon chili powder
- 1/2 teaspoon cumin
- 1/4 cup low-fat shredded cheese

Directions:

1. Preheat oven to 375°F (190°C).

2. In a bowl, mix quinoa, black beans, corn, tomato, cilantro, chili powder, and cumin.

3. Stuff each bell pepper with the quinoa mixture and place in a baking dish.

4. Top with shredded cheese and bake for 25 minutes.

Nutrition per serving: Calories: 250 | Total Fat: 3g | Sat Fat: 1g | Carbs: 45g | Fiber: 10g | Protein: 13g | Sodium: 300mg

5. Grilled Veggie and Hummus Wrap

Preparation Time: 15 Minutes | Cook Time: 10 Minutes | Makes 4 Servings

Ingredients:

- 4 whole wheat tortillas
- 1 zucchini, sliced
- 1 yellow squash, sliced
- 1 red bell pepper, sliced
- 1 tablespoon olive oil
- 1 cup hummus
- Salt and pepper to taste

Directions:

1. Toss zucchini, squash, and bell pepper with olive oil, salt, and pepper.

2. Grill vegetables until tender, about 5 minutes per side.

3. Spread each tortilla with hummus, add grilled vegetables, roll up, and serve.

Nutrition per serving: Calories: 280 | Total Fat: 10g | Sat Fat: 1g | Carbs: 42g | Fiber: 8g | Protein: 10g | Sodium: 400mg

6. Avocado and Egg Salad Sandwich

Preparation Time: 10 Minutes | Makes 4 Servings

Ingredients:

- 4 hard-boiled eggs, peeled and chopped
- 1 ripe avocado, mashed
- 1 tablespoon lemon juice
- 1/4 teaspoon paprika
- Salt and pepper to taste
- 8 slices whole grain bread
- Lettuce leaves

Directions:

1. In a bowl, mix chopped eggs, mashed avocado, lemon juice, paprika, salt, and pepper.

2. Spread the mixture onto 4 slices of bread, top with lettuce, and cover with the remaining bread slices.

Nutrition per serving: Calories: 300 | Total Fat: 12g | Sat Fat: 3g | Carbs: 35g | Fiber: 7g | Protein: 13g | Sodium: 400mg

7. Greek Yogurt Chicken Salad

Preparation Time: 15 Minutes | Makes 4 Servings

Ingredients:

- 2 cups cooked chicken breast, shredded
- 1/2 cup Greek yogurt
- 1/4 cup celery, chopped
- 1/4 cup grapes, halved
- 1/4 cup almonds, sliced
- 1 tablespoon honey
- Salt and pepper to taste
- 4 cups mixed salad greens

Directions:

1. In a bowl, mix chicken, Greek yogurt, celery, grapes, almonds, and honey.

2. Season with salt and pepper.

3. Serve over a bed of mixed salad greens.

Nutrition per serving: Calories: 230 | Total Fat: 6g | Sat Fat: 1g | Carbs: 14g | Fiber: 2g | Protein: 30g | Sodium: 150mg

9.Lentil and Vegetable Soup

Preparation Time: 15 Minutes | Cook Time: 30 Minutes | Makes 6 Servings

Ingredients:

- 1 tablespoon olive oil
- 1 onion, chopped
- 2 carrots, diced
- 2 celery stalks, diced
- 1 garlic clove, minced
- 1 cup dried lentils, rinsed
- 4 cups vegetable broth
- 1 can (14.5 ounces) diced tomatoes
- 1 teaspoon thyme
- Salt and pepper to taste

Directions:

1. Heat olive oil in a large pot over medium heat. Add onion, carrots, celery, and garlic, and sauté for 5 minutes.

2. Add lentils, broth, tomatoes, and thyme. Bring to a boil, reduce heat, and simmer for 30 minutes.

3. Season with salt and pepper, and serve.

Nutrition per serving: Calories: 180 | Total Fat: 2g | Sat Fat: 0g | Carbs: 30g | Fiber: 10g | Protein: 10g | Sodium: 300mg

11. Roasted Vegetable and Goat Cheese Frittata

Preparation Time: 15 Minutes | Cook Time: 25 Minutes | Makes 4 Servings

Ingredients:

- 6 eggs
- 1/4 cup milk
- 1 cup roasted vegetables (bell peppers, zucchini, onions)
- 1/4 cup goat cheese, crumbled
- Salt and pepper to taste
- 1 tablespoon olive oil

Directions:

1. Preheat oven to 375°F (190°C).

2. In a bowl, whisk together eggs, milk, salt, and pepper.

3. Heat olive oil in an ovenproof skillet over medium heat. Add roasted vegetables and pour the egg mixture over the top.

4. Sprinkle with goat cheese and cook for 5 minutes without stirring.

5. Transfer skillet to oven and bake for 20 minutes, or until frittata is set.

Nutrition per serving: Calories: 210 | Total Fat: 13g | Sat Fat: 5g | Carbs: 8g | Fiber: 2g

10 Wholesome Dinner Recipes

1. Quinoa and Black Bean Stuffed Peppers

Preparation Time: 20 Minutes | Total Time: 1 Hour | Makes 6 Servings

Ingredients:

- 6 large bell peppers, tops cut away and seeds removed
- 1 cup quinoa, rinsed
- 2 cups vegetable broth
- 1 can (15 ounces) black beans, drained and rinsed
- 1 cup corn kernels (fresh or frozen)
- 1/2 cup chopped red onion
- 1/2 cup finely chopped cilantro
- 1 teaspoon ground cumin
- 1 teaspoon smoked paprika
- 1/2 teaspoon garlic powder
- Salt and pepper to taste
- 1 cup grated low-fat Monterey Jack cheese
- Fresh lime wedges for serving

Directions:

1. Preheat the oven to 350°F.

2. In a medium saucepan, combine quinoa and vegetable broth. Bring to a boil, then reduce heat to low, cover, and simmer for 15 minutes or until quinoa is cooked and liquid is absorbed.

3. In a large bowl, mix cooked quinoa, black beans, corn, red onion, cilantro, cumin, smoked paprika, garlic powder, salt, and pepper.

4. Arrange the bell peppers in a baking dish. Spoon the quinoa mixture into each pepper cavity.

5. Sprinkle the tops with grated cheese.

6. Cover the baking dish with aluminum foil and bake for 30 minutes. Then, remove the foil and bake for an additional 10 minutes, or until the peppers are tender and the cheese is melted and slightly browned.

7. Serve the stuffed peppers hot, with fresh lime wedges on the side.

Nutrition per serving: Calories 256 | Total Fat 6g | Sat Fat 2g | Carbs 40g | Fiber 9g | Protein 13g | Sodium 307mg

2. Lemon Garlic Shrimp and Asparagus

Preparation Time: 10 Minutes | Total Time: 20 Minutes | Makes 4 Servings

Ingredients:

- 1 pound large shrimp, peeled and deveined
- 2 tablespoons olive oil
- 4 cloves garlic, minced
- Juice of 1 lemon
- 1 pound asparagus, ends trimmed
- Salt and pepper to taste
- Red pepper flakes (optional)

Directions:

1. In a large skillet, heat olive oil over medium heat.

2. Add garlic and sauté for 1 minute.

3. Add shrimp and cook until pink, about 3-4 minutes per side.

4. Add asparagus, lemon juice, salt, pepper, and red pepper flakes. Cook until asparagus is tender, about 4-5 minutes.

5. Serve hot.

Nutrition per serving: Calories 190 | Total Fat 8g | Sat Fat 1g | Carbs 6g | Fiber 2g | Protein 24g | Sodium 210mg

3. Turkey and Spinach Stuffed Sweet Potatoes

Preparation Time: 15 Minutes | Total Time: 1 Hour | Makes 4 Servings

Ingredients:

- 4 medium sweet potatoes
- 1 pound lean ground turkey
- 1 teaspoon olive oil
- 1 small onion, chopped
- 2 cloves garlic, minced
- 2 cups fresh spinach
- 1 teaspoon paprika
- Salt and pepper to taste
- 1/4 cup low-fat feta cheese, crumbled

Directions:

1. Preheat the oven to 400°F.

2. Pierce sweet potatoes with a fork and bake until tender, about 45 minutes.

3. In a skillet, heat olive oil over medium heat. Add onion and garlic, sautéing until soft.

4. Add ground turkey, cooking until browned.

5. Stir in spinach, paprika, salt, and pepper, cooking until spinach wilts.

6. Cut sweet potatoes in half lengthwise, and scoop out a bit of the flesh to create a "bowl".

7. Fill each sweet potato with the turkey mixture and top with feta cheese.

8. Serve warm.

Nutrition per serving: Calories 290 | Total Fat 6g | Sat Fat 2g | Carbs 35g | Fiber 6g | Protein 24g | Sodium 320mg

4. Mediterranean Chickpea Salad

Preparation Time: 15 Minutes | Total Time: 15 Minutes | Makes 4 Servings

Ingredients:

- 2 cans (15 ounces each) chickpeas, drained and rinsed
- 1 cucumber, diced
- 1 bell pepper, diced
- 1/2 red onion, finely chopped
- 1/2 cup cherry tomatoes, halved
- 1/4 cup chopped fresh parsley
- Juice of 1 lemon
- 2 tablespoons olive oil
- Salt and pepper to taste
- 1/4 cup crumbled low-fat feta cheese

Directions:

1. In a large bowl, combine chickpeas, cucumber, bell pepper, onion, tomatoes, and parsley.

2. In a small bowl, whisk together lemon juice, olive oil, salt, and pepper.

3. Pour dressing over salad and toss to coat.

4. Sprinkle with feta cheese before serving.

Nutrition per serving: Calories 265 | Total Fat 10g | Sat Fat 2g | Carbs 36g | Fiber 10g | Protein 11g | Sodium 400mg

5. Zucchini Noodles with Pesto Chicken

Preparation Time: 10 Minutes | Total Time: 20 Minutes | Makes 4 Servings

Ingredients:

- 2 large zucchinis, spiralized into noodles
- 1 pound boneless, skinless chicken breasts, cut into strips
- 1 tablespoon olive oil
- Salt and pepper to taste
- 1/2 cup homemade or store-bought low-fat pesto
- Cherry tomatoes for garnish (optional)

Directions:

1. In a skillet, heat olive oil over medium heat.

2. Season chicken with salt and pepper and cook until golden and cooked through, about 5-6 minutes per side.

3. Toss zucchini noodles with pesto sauce in a large bowl.

4. Add cooked chicken to the zucchini noodles and toss to combine.

5. Garnish with cherry tomatoes if desired and serve.

Nutrition per serving: Calories 250 | Total Fat 13g | Sat Fat 2g | Carbs 6g | Fiber 2g | Protein 28g | Sodium 320mg

6. Baked Salmon with Dill and Lemon

Preparation Time: 5 Minutes | Total Time: 20 Minutes | Makes 4 Servings

Ingredients:

- 4 salmon fillets (4 ounces each)
- 2 tablespoons olive oil
- Juice of 1 lemon
- 2 tablespoons fresh dill, chopped
- Salt and pepper to taste
- Lemon slices for garnish

Directions:

1. Preheat oven to 400°F.

2. Place salmon on a baking sheet lined with parchment paper.

3. Drizzle olive oil and lemon juice over the salmon. Season with salt, pepper, and dill.

4. Bake for 12-15 minutes or until salmon flakes easily with a fork.

5. Serve garnished with lemon slices.

Nutrition per serving: Calories 240 | Total Fat 15g | Sat Fat 2g | Carbs 1g | Fiber 0g | Protein 23g | Sodium 60mg

7. Cauliflower Fried Rice with Vegetables

Preparation Time: 10 Minutes | Total Time: 20 Minutes | Makes 4 Servings

Ingredients:

- 1 head cauliflower, grated into "rice"
- 1 tablespoon sesame oil
- 1 small onion, diced
- 1 cup frozen peas and carrots
- 2 cloves garlic, minced
- 2 eggs, lightly beaten
- 2 tablespoons low-sodium soy sauce
- Green onions for garnish

Directions:

1. Heat sesame oil in a large skillet over medium heat.

2. Add onion and garlic, sautéing until translucent.

3. Stir in peas and carrots, cooking until heated through.

4. Move vegetables to one side of the skillet and add eggs to the other side, scrambling until cooked.

5. Add cauliflower rice and soy sauce, mix everything, and cook for 5 minutes.

6. Garnish with green onions before serving.

Nutrition per serving: Calories 150 | Total Fat 7g | Sat Fat 1.5g | Carbs 15g | Fiber 5g | Protein 9g | Sodium 320mg

8. Spicy Lentil Soup Preparation Time: 15 Minutes | Total Time: 45 Minutes | Makes 6 Servings

Ingredients:

- 1 cup dried lentils, rinsed
- 1 tablespoon olive oil
- 1 onion, chopped
- 2 carrots, diced
- 2 stalks celery, diced
- 3 cloves garlic, minced
- 1 teaspoon ground cumin
- 1/2 teaspoon chili powder
- 6 cups vegetable broth
- Salt and pepper to taste
- Fresh parsley for garnish

Directions:

1. In a large pot, heat olive oil over medium heat.

2. Add onion, carrots, celery, and garlic. Cook until vegetables are tender.

3. Stir in cumin and chili powder.

4. Add lentils and vegetable broth. Bring to a boil, then reduce heat and simmer for 30 minutes or until lentils are tender.

5. Season with salt and pepper.

6. Garnish with fresh parsley before serving.

Nutrition per serving: Calories 190 | Total Fat 3g | Sat Fat 0.5g | Carbs 30g | Fiber 10g | Protein 12g | Sodium 400mg

9. Grilled Chicken and Vegetable Kabobs

Preparation Time: 15 Minutes (plus marinating) | Total Time: 30 Minutes | Makes 4 Servings

Ingredients:

- 1 pound boneless, skinless chicken breasts, cut into cubes
- 2 zucchinis, sliced into rounds
- 1 bell pepper, cut into chunks
- 1 red onion, cut into chunks

For the marinade:

- 1/4 cup olive oil

- 3 tablespoons lemon juice

- 1 teaspoon garlic powder

- 1 teaspoon dried oregano

- Salt and pepper to taste

Directions:

1. In a bowl, whisk together all marinade ingredients.

2. Add chicken to the marinade, cover, and refrigerate for at least 30 minutes.

3. Preheat the grill to medium-high heat.

4. Thread chicken, zucchini, bell pepper, and onion onto skewers.

5. Grill for 10-15 minutes, turning occasionally, until chicken is cooked through.

6. Serve hot.

Nutrition per serving: Calories 290 | Total Fat 15g | Sat Fat 2.5g | Carbs 8g | Fiber 2g | Protein 30g | Sodium 200mg

10. Spicy Chickpea and Spinach Stew

Preparation Time: 15 Minutes | Total Time: 40 Minutes | Makes 4 Servings

Ingredients:

- 2 tablespoons olive oil
- 1 large onion, chopped
- 3 cloves garlic, minced
- 1 teaspoon ground cumin
- 1 teaspoon ground coriander
- 1/2 teaspoon cayenne pepper (adjust to taste)
- 1 can (14.5 ounces) diced tomatoes
- 1 can (15 ounces) chickpeas, drained and rinsed
- 2 cups vegetable broth
- 4 cups fresh spinach leaves
- Salt and pepper to taste
- 2 tablespoons fresh lemon juice
- Fresh cilantro, chopped, for garnish

Directions:

1. Heat olive oil in a large pot over medium heat. Add the onion and garlic, sautéing until the onion is translucent, about 5 minutes.

2. Stir in cumin, coriander, and cayenne pepper, cooking for another minute until fragrant.

3. Add the diced tomatoes (with their juice), chickpeas, and vegetable broth. Bring to a boil, then reduce heat and simmer for 20 minutes.

4. Add the spinach to the pot, stirring until it wilts, about 3 minutes.

5. Season with salt and pepper, and stir in the lemon juice.

6. Serve hot, garnished with fresh cilantro.

Nutrition per serving: Calories 210 | Total Fat 7g | Sat Fat 1g | Carbs 30g | Fiber 8g | Protein 8g | Sodium 410mg

10 Low-Calorie Snack Recipes

1. Cucumber and Hummus Rolls

Preparation Time: 10 Minutes | Total Time: 10 Minutes | Makes 6 Servings

Ingredients:

- 2 large cucumbers, thinly sliced lengthwise
- 1 cup hummus
- ½ red bell pepper, finely diced
- ¼ cup Kalamata olives, chopped
- 1 tablespoon lemon juice
- Salt and pepper to taste

Directions:

- Lay cucumber slices on a flat surface. Spread a thin layer of hummus on each slice.

- Sprinkle red bell pepper and olives on top. Drizzle with lemon juice, and season with salt and pepper.

- Roll each cucumber slice tightly and secure it with a toothpick.

Nutrition per serving: Calories 70 | Total Fat 4g | Sat Fat 0.5g | Carbs 8g | Fibre 2g | Protein 3g | Sodium 130mg

2. Spicy Roasted Chickpeas

Preparation Time: 5 Minutes | Total Time: 40 Minutes | Makes 4 Servings

Ingredients:

- 1 can (15 oz) chickpeas, drained and rinsed
- 1 tablespoon olive oil
- ½ teaspoon smoked paprika
- ¼ teaspoon cayenne pepper
- Salt to taste

Directions:

- Preheat oven to 400°F. Pat chickpeas dry with a towel.

- In a bowl, toss chickpeas with olive oil, paprika, cayenne, and salt.

- Spread on a baking sheet in a single layer and roast for 30-35 minutes, stirring occasionally, until crispy.

Nutrition per serving: Calories 120 | Total Fat 4g | Sat Fat 0.5g | Carbs 16g | Fibre 5g | Protein 5g | Sodium 200mg

3. Greek Yogurt and Berry Parfait

Preparation Time: 5 Minutes | Total Time: 5 Minutes | Makes 1 Serving

Ingredients:

- 1 cup non-fat Greek yogurt
- ½ cup mixed berries (strawberries, blueberries, raspberries)
- 1 tablespoon honey
- 1 tablespoon chopped nuts (optional)

Directions:

- In a glass, layer Greek yogurt and mixed berries.

- Drizzle with honey and top with chopped nuts if desired.

Nutrition per serving: Calories 150 | Total Fat 1g | Sat Fat 0g | Carbs 22g | Fibre 3g | Protein 14g | Sodium 50mg

4. Veggie Sticks with Avocado Dip

Preparation Time: 10 Minutes | Total Time: 10 Minutes | Makes 4 Servings

Ingredients:

- 1 ripe avocado, mashed
- 1 tablespoon lime juice
- 1 garlic clove, minced
- Salt and pepper to taste
- Assorted veggie sticks (carrots, celery, bell peppers)

Directions:

- In a bowl, mix mashed avocado with lime juice, garlic, salt, and pepper.

- Serve with assorted veggie sticks for dipping.

Nutrition per serving: Calories 80 | Total Fat 6g | Sat Fat 1g | Carbs 6g | Fibre 4g | Protein 2g | Sodium 60mg

5. Apple Peanut Butter Slices

Preparation Time: 5 Minutes | Total Time: 5 Minutes | Makes 2 Servings

Ingredients:

- 1 large apple, cored and sliced

- 2 tablespoons natural peanut butter

Directions:

- Spread peanut butter evenly on apple slices.

Nutrition per serving: Calories 165 | Total Fat 8g | Sat Fat 1.5g | Carbs 22g | Fibre 4g | Protein 4g | Sodium 75mg

6. Baked Sweet Potato Fries

Preparation Time: 10 Minutes | Total Time: 30 Minutes | Makes 4 Servings

Ingredients:

• 2 large sweet potatoes, peeled and cut into fries

• 1 tablespoon olive oil

• ½ teaspoon paprika

• Salt to taste

Directions:

• Preheat oven to 425°F. Toss sweet potato fries with olive oil, paprika, and salt.

• Spread on a baking sheet in a single layer and bake for 20 minutes, turning halfway through.

Nutrition per serving: Calories 110 | Total Fat 3.5g | Sat Fat 0.5g | Carbs 18g | Fibre 3g | Protein 2g | Sodium 120mg

7. Zucchini Chips

Preparation Time: 10 Minutes | Total Time: 2 Hours | Makes 4 Servings

Ingredients:

• 2 large zucchinis, thinly sliced

• 1 tablespoon olive oil

• Salt to taste

Directions:

• Preheat oven to 225°F. Toss zucchini slices with olive oil and salt.

• Arrange slices on a baking sheet lined with parchment paper and bake for 1½-2 hours until crispy.

Nutrition per serving: Calories 60 | Total Fat 3.5g | Sat Fat 0.5g | Carbs 6g | Fibre 2g | Protein 2g | Sodium 10mg

8. Mini Bell Pepper Boats

Preparation Time: 15 Minutes | Total Time: 15 Minutes | Makes 6 Servings

Ingredients:

- 12 mini bell peppers, halved and seeded
- 1 cup cottage cheese
- 2 tablespoons chopped chives
- 1 tablespoon lemon juice
- Salt and pepper to taste

Directions:

- In a bowl, mix cottage cheese with chives, lemon juice, salt, and pepper.
- Spoon the mixture into each bell pepper half.

Nutrition per serving: Calories 50 | Total Fat 0.5g | Sat Fat 0g | Carbs 6g | Fibre 2g | Protein 6g | Sodium 180mg

9. Frozen Banana Bites

Preparation Time: 15 Minutes | Total Time: 2 Hours 15 Minutes | Makes 4 Servings

Ingredients:

• 2 bananas, sliced

• ¼ cup dark chocolate chips, melted

• 1 tablespoon chopped nuts (optional)

Directions:

• Dip banana slices in melted chocolate and sprinkle with nuts if desired.

• Place on a parchment-lined tray and freeze for 2 hours.

Nutrition per serving: Calories 100 | Total Fat 3g | Sat Fat 1.5g | Carbs 18g | Fibre 2g | Protein 1g | Sodium 0mg

10. Edamame with Sea Salt

Preparation Time: 5 Minutes | Total Time: 5 Minutes | Makes 4 Servings

Ingredients:

- 2 cups frozen edamame, thawed
- 1 teaspoon sea salt

Directions:

- Sprinkle edamame with sea salt and serve.

Nutrition per serving: Calories 120 | Total Fat 5g | Sat Fat 0.5g | Carbs 10g | Fibre 5g | Protein 11g | Sodium 290mg

10 Invigorating Drink Recipes

1. Green Tea Citrus Blast

Preparation Time: 10 Minutes | Total Time: 15 Minutes | Makes 4 Servings

Ingredients:

- 4 bags of green tea
- 4 cups boiling water
- 2 oranges, juiced
- 1 lemon, juiced
- 1 tablespoon grated ginger
- 2 tablespoons honey (optional)
- Fresh mint leaves, for garnish
- Ice cubes

Directions:

1. Steep the green tea bags in boiling water for 5 minutes. Remove tea bags and allow the tea to cool to room temperature.

2. In a large pitcher, combine the cooled green tea, orange juice, lemon juice, and grated ginger.

3. If desired, add honey to sweeten and stir well.

4. Refrigerate the mixture for at least an hour to chill.

5. Serve over ice cubes in glasses, garnished with fresh mint leaves.

Nutrition per serving: Calories 35 (without honey) | Total Fat 0g | Sat Fat 0g | Carbs 9g | Fibre 1g | Protein 0g | Sodium 2mg

2. Berry Protein Smoothie

Preparation Time: 5 Minutes | Total Time: 7 Minutes | Makes 2 Servings

Ingredients:

- 1 cup mixed berries (strawberries, blueberries, raspberries)
- 1 banana
- 1 cup spinach leaves
- 1 scoop protein powder (vanilla or unflavored)
- 1 cup almond milk
- Ice cubes

Directions:

- Blend all ingredients until smooth. Serve immediately.

Nutrition per serving: Calories 150 | Total Fat 2g | Sat Fat 0g | Carbs 22g | Fiber 4g | Protein 10g | Sodium 80mg

3. Cucumber Mint Refresher

Preparation Time: 10 Minutes | Total Time: 15 Minutes | Makes 4 Servings

Ingredients:

- 1 large cucumber, peeled and sliced
- fresh mint leaves
- 2 tablespoons lime juice
- 1-liter sparkling water
- Ice cubes

Directions:

- Blend cucumber, mint, and lime juice. Strain and mix with sparkling water. Serve over ice.

Nutrition per serving: Calories 12 | Total Fat 0g | Sat Fat 0g | Carbs 3g | Fiber 1g | Protein 0g | Sodium 2mg

4. Spiced Apple Detox Tea

Preparation Time: 5 Minutes | Total Time: 20 Minutes | Makes 4 Servings

Ingredients:

- 4 cups water
- 2 cinnamon sticks
- 4 cloves
- 2 apples, sliced
- 1 tablespoon honey (optional)

Directions:

- Simmer water with cinnamon, cloves, and apples for 15 minutes. Strain and add honey if desired. Serve hot.

Nutrition per serving: Calories 30 (without honey) | Total Fat 0g | Sat Fat 0g | Carbs 8g | Fiber 1g | Protein 0g | Sodium 0mg

5. Ginger Lemonade

Preparation Time: 10 Minutes | Total Time: 15 Minutes | Makes 4 Servings

Ingredients:

- 4 cups water
- 1/2 cup lemon juice
- 2 tablespoons grated ginger
- 2 tablespoons honey (optional)

Directions:

- Combine water, lemon juice, and ginger. Sweeten with honey if desired. Serve chilled over ice.

Nutrition per serving: Calories 25 (without honey) | Total Fat 0g | Sat Fat 0g | Carbs 7g | Fiber 0g | Protein 0g | Sodium 1mg

6. Carrot and Orange Boost

Preparation Time: 10 Minutes | Total Time: 15 Minutes | Makes 2 Servings

Ingredients:

- 3 large carrots, peeled
- 2 oranges, juiced
- 1-inch piece of ginger, peeled

Directions:

- Juice all ingredients and stir. Serve immediately over ice.

Nutrition per serving: Calories 120 | Total Fat 0.5g | Sat Fat 0g | Carbs 28g | Fiber 7g | Protein 2g | Sodium 70mg

7. Tropical Turmeric Smoothie

Preparation Time: 5 Minutes | Total Time: 7 Minutes | Makes 2 Servings

Ingredients:

- 1 cup pineapple chunks
- 1 banana
- 1/2 teaspoon turmeric powder
- 1 cup coconut water
- Ice cubes

Directions:

- Blend all ingredients until smooth. Serve immediately.

Nutrition per serving: Calories 120 | Total Fat 0.5g | Sat Fat 0g | Carbs 30g | Fiber 3g | Protein 1g | Sodium 40mg

8. Watermelon Hydrator

Preparation Time: 5 Minutes | Total Time: 7 Minutes | Makes 4 Servings

Ingredients:

- 4 cups watermelon, cubed
- Juice of 1 lime
- 1 cup coconut water
- Ice cubes

Directions:

- Blend watermelon, lime juice, and coconut water. Serve over ice.

Nutrition per serving: Calories 50 | Total Fat 0g | Sat Fat 0g | Carbs 13g | Fiber 1g | Protein 1g | Sodium 25mg

9. Beetroot and Berry Fusion

Preparation Time: 10 Minutes | Total Time: 15 Minutes | Makes 2 Servings

Ingredients:

- 1 small beetroot, peeled
- 1 cup mixed berries
- 1 apple, cored
- 1 cup water or coconut water

Directions:

- Juice all ingredients and stir well. Serve chilled.

Nutrition per serving: Calories 90 | Total Fat 0g | Sat Fat 0g | Carbs 22g | Fiber 4g | Protein 1g | Sodium 30mg

10. Almond Milk Chai

Preparation Time: 5 Minutes | Total Time: 10 Minutes | Makes 2 Servings

Ingredients:

- 2 cups almond milk
- 1 cinnamon stick
- 2 cardamom pods
- 1-star anise
- 1 tablespoon black tea leaves or 2 tea bags
- 1 tablespoon honey (optional)

Directions:

- Simmer almond milk with spices and tea for 5 minutes. Strain and add honey if desired. Serve hot.

Nutrition per serving: Calories 60 (without honey) | Total Fat 2.5g | Sat Fat 0g | Carbs 8g | Fiber 1g | Protein 1g | Sodium 160mg

CHAPTER 5: INTEGRATING EXERCISE INTO YOUR ROUTINE

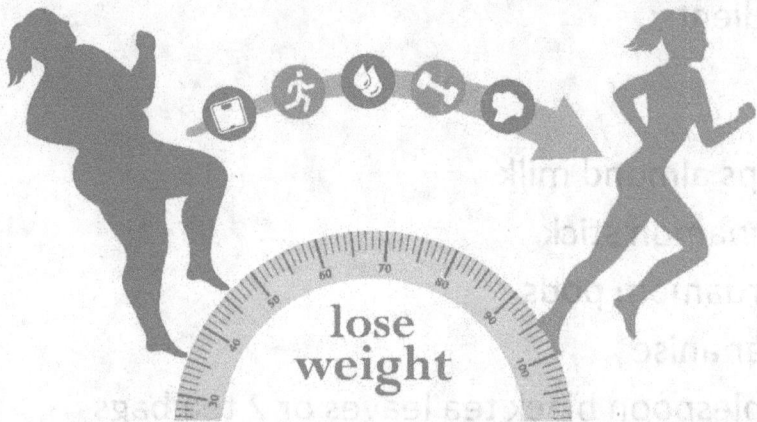

In our journey towards a healthier self, the symbiosis of diet and exercise forms the cornerstone of effective weight loss. While the previous chapters have laid a strong foundation on the dietary aspects, it's now time to elevate our focus to the physical dimension of our wellness journey. This chapter, "Integrating Exercise into Your Routine," is designed not just as a guide, but as a gentle companion in your journey towards integrating exercise into your life, harmoniously balancing it with the nutritional insights garnered from earlier sections.

Easy Exercises for Beginners

Embarking on an exercise regimen can be daunting, especially for beginners. The key lies in starting with simplicity and progressing steadily. Let's explore exercises that are beginner-friendly yet effective in complementing the dietary strategies discussed previously.

1. **Walking:** A quintessential exercise, walking is an excellent start for beginners. It's low impact, easily adjustable in intensity, and can be done almost anywhere. A daily brisk walk can significantly boost your metabolism, aiding in weight loss.

2. **Yoga:** With its roots in holistic wellness, yoga is more than physical exercise. It's a blend of physical postures, breathing techniques, and meditation, making it an ideal exercise for those seeking a gentle yet effective workout. Yoga can improve flexibility, strength, and mindfulness, all crucial for a balanced weight loss journey.

3. **Strength Training with Body Weight:** Exercises like squats, lunges, and push-ups, use your body weight to build strength. They are pivotal in building lean muscle mass, which in turn accelerates your metabolism.

4. **Swimming:** If you have access to a pool, swimming is a fantastic low-impact exercise. It's excellent for

cardiovascular health and engages multiple muscle groups without stressing the joints.

5. **Cycling:** Whether outdoor or on a stationary bike, cycling is an enjoyable and effective way to improve cardiovascular health and burn calories.

Balancing Diet and Exercise

The true art of weight loss is in the balance of diet and exercise. Neither can be effective in isolation. This book has already laid a nutritional foundation – now, let's integrate it with physical activity.

1. **Understand Your Body's Needs:** Just as we've learned about personalized dietary needs, understand that exercise routines also need personalization. Listen to your body and adjust the intensity and type of exercise accordingly.

2. **Consistency Over Intensity:** It's more beneficial to exercise moderately but regularly, rather than pursuing intense workouts sporadically. Consistency helps in building long-term habits and ensures sustained weight loss.

3. **Nutrition and Workout Synergy:** Post-exercise, your body needs nutrients for recovery. Plan your meals such that they complement your workout routine – like a

protein-rich meal after strength training or a carbohydrate-rich meal after endurance activities.

4. **Rest and Recovery:** Rest days are crucial. They allow your body to recover, preventing burnout and injuries. A balanced approach to diet and exercise includes understanding the importance of rest.

In conclusion, integrating exercise into your routine isn't just about physical activity; it's about creating a harmonious relationship between your body's nutritional and physical needs. As you advance through this chapter, remember that each step forward is a step towards a healthier, more vibrant you. The combination of a well-structured diet and a thoughtfully integrated exercise regime is the secret to not just losing weight, but embracing a lifestyle of sustained wellness.

CHAPTER 6: OVERCOMING CHALLENGES

In the journey of weight loss, encountering hurdles is not just a possibility, it's an inevitability. The true test of resilience isn't in the uninterrupted success but in how we navigate the rough waters. This chapter delves into two of the most common challenges faced by individuals on their weight loss journey: dealing with plateaus and maintaining motivation.

Dealing with Plateaus

A weight loss plateau is a phase where the scale refuses to budge despite your efforts. It's not just a hurdle; it's a natural part of the body's response to weight loss. Initially, as you start to change your diet and exercise routine, the body responds quickly. Over time, however, the body adapts to these changes, and weight loss can slow down or stall.

Understanding the science behind plateaus is crucial. As you lose weight, your body requires fewer calories to maintain its new, lighter self. This reduced caloric need can lead to a plateau if your calorie intake and expenditure don't adjust accordingly. It's a sign that your body is becoming more efficient, a positive indicator of progress.

To break through a plateau, consider the following strategies:

1. **Reevaluate Your Caloric Needs**: As your body changes, so do your caloric requirements. Adjust your diet to align with your current metabolic needs.

2. **Mix Up Your Exercise Routine**: Introduce new exercises or increase the intensity of your current workouts to challenge your body in new ways.

3. **Monitor and Adjust Your Eating Habits**: Keep a close eye on your dietary habits. Sometimes, small, unnoticed calories can creep in and affect your progress.

4. **Focus on Body Composition, Not Just Weight**: Remember, muscle is denser than fat. Use measurements and how your clothes fit as additional indicators of your progress.

Maintaining Motivation

Motivation is the fuel for your weight loss journey. However, keeping the flame of motivation burning can be challenging, especially when progress seems slow or obstacles arise.

Here are strategies to help maintain your motivation:

1. **Set Realistic and Achievable Goals**: Unrealistic goals can lead to disappointment. Break down your main goal into smaller, manageable milestones and celebrate each achievement.

2.   **Find a Support System**: Surround yourself with people who understand and support your goals. Joining a weight loss group or finding a workout buddy can provide encouragement and accountability.

3.   **Keep a Progress Journal**: Documenting your journey, including the ups and downs, can provide perspective and help you see how far you've come.

4.   **Stay Flexible and Patient**: Be prepared to adjust your plans as needed. Patience is vital; weight loss is a marathon, not a sprint.

5.   **Remind Yourself of the 'Why'**: Regularly remind yourself why you started this journey. Whether it's for health, confidence, or another personal reason, keeping your 'why' in focus can reignite motivation.

Remember, overcoming challenges in your weight loss journey is not just about altering strategies, but also about strengthening your mindset. Embrace plateaus as opportunities for learning and growth, and keep your motivational flame alive by focusing on your goals, celebrating small victories, and reminding yourself of the reasons behind your journey. By understanding and applying these principles, you can navigate through these challenges and continue towards your weight loss goals with confidence and resilience.

CHAPTER 7: CONCLUSION
LONG-TERM SUCCESS

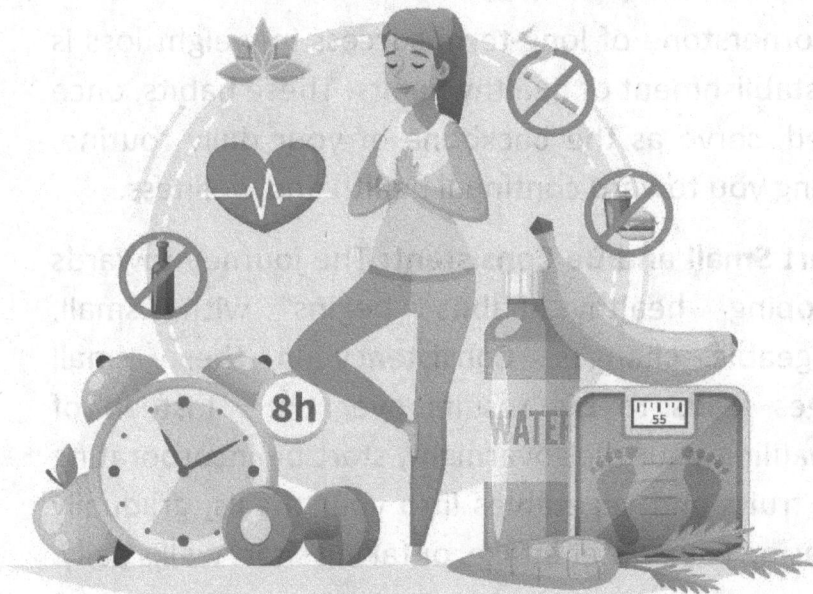

HEALTHY LIFESTYLE

In the quest for weight loss, the true victory lies not in the shedding of pounds alone, but in the mastery of long-term health and wellness. This journey, often riddled with challenges and setbacks, calls for more than just a temporary fix or a quick diet plan. It demands a transformation of lifestyle, a redefinition of habits, and a steadfast commitment to maintaining a state of health and fitness. In this chapter, we delve deep into the art of sustaining this triumphant state, guiding you through the labyrinth of developing healthy habits and staying fit, not just for days or months, but for a lifetime.

Developing Healthy Habits

The cornerstone of long-term success in weight loss is the establishment of healthy habits. These habits, once formed, serve as the backbone of your daily routine, steering you toward continual health and wellness.

1. Start Small and Be Consistent: The journey towards developing healthy habits begins with small, manageable changes. Consistency in these small changes leads to big results over time. Instead of overhauling your diet overnight, start by incorporating more fruits and vegetables into your meals, gradually increasing your water intake, or taking short walks daily.

2. Understand Your Body's Needs: Each body is unique, and understanding what works best for you is crucial. Pay attention to how different foods and exercises affect your body and mind. Tailoring your diet and exercise routine to suit your individual needs is more sustainable in the long run.

3. Set Realistic Goals: Unrealistic goals can lead to frustration and demotivation. Set achievable targets, such as losing a certain amount of weight over a reasonable period or gradually increasing your exercise intensity.

4. Mindful Eating: Develop a habit of mindful eating. This means being fully present during meals, savoring each bite, and listening to your body's hunger and fullness cues. This practice helps in avoiding overeating and makes meals more enjoyable and satisfying.

5. Consistent Sleep Patterns: Adequate and regular sleep is vital. Lack of sleep can disrupt metabolism and lead to weight gain. Establish a consistent sleep schedule to improve your overall health.

Staying Healthy and Fit

Maintaining health and fitness is an ongoing process that requires perseverance and adaptation. As you evolve, so should your approach to staying healthy.

1. Embrace Variety: Avoid monotony in your diet and exercise routine. Experiment with different healthy foods and recipes to keep your meals exciting. Similarly, vary your physical activities to engage different muscle groups and keep the exercise interesting.

2. Continuous Learning: Stay informed about the latest research in nutrition and fitness. Knowledge empowers you to make better choices and adapt your habits as needed.

3. Regular Health Check-ups: Regular check-ups with healthcare professionals can help in the early detection of any health issues and ensure you're on the right track.

4. Mental Health: Never underestimate the power of mental well-being in your weight loss journey. Practices like meditation, yoga, or simply taking time to relax and de-stress contribute significantly to your overall health.

5. Building a Support System: Surround yourself with people who support and motivate you. Joining communities, whether online or in-person, where members share similar goals can provide encouragement and valuable tips.

In conclusion, long-term success in weight loss is not just about reaching a target weight, but about creating a lifestyle that naturally supports your health and fitness goals. By developing healthy habits and focusing on maintaining these practices, you set yourself up for a lifetime of health, vitality, and happiness. Remember, your health journey is continuous, and each step you take is a step towards a more fulfilled and vibrant life.

ADDITIONAL RESOURCES

Books and Publications:

1.   **"The China Study" by T. Colin Campbell and Thomas M. Campbell:** Explores the relationship between the consumption of animal products and chronic illnesses.

2.   **"Eat to Live" by Joel Fuhrman, M.D.:** Focuses on nutrient-dense, plant-rich eating for health and weight loss.

3.   **"The Blue Zones" by Dan Buettner:** Investigates communities worldwide where people live longer and healthier lives.

4.   **"Self Heal by Design"** by Barbara O'Neill: It embraces natural health principles and holistic practices for self-healing and wellness.

Online Resources:

1.   **NutritionFacts.org:** A non-profit website providing the latest in nutrition-related research.

2.   **MyFitnessPal:** An app for tracking diet and exercise, useful for understanding caloric intake and expenditure.

3.   **Whole30:** A resource for whole food-based diet planning, focusing on eliminating processed foods.

Community Support:

1.   **Local Cooking Classes:** Many communities offer healthy cooking classes focusing on weight loss and nutritious meal preparation.

2.   **Online Forums and Groups:** Platforms like Reddit and Facebook have various groups dedicated to weight loss, diet, and fitness where individuals can share experiences and advice.